WEIGHT WATCHERS INSTANT POT COOKBOOK

Delicious Smartpoints Recipes, Quick To Prepare and Faster Weight Loss

By

William WW

Table of Contents

Dinner: Baked Chicken Quesadilla Casserole Smartpoints (Freestyle): 6

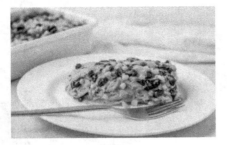

Growing up, "quesadillas" were one of many things my sister and I realized we could "cook" all by ourselves in the microwave.

Our recipe was simple: Two tortillas and whatever kind of cheese my mom had in the fridge. We just popped it all in the microwave until it was melted and garnished it with a dollop of sour cream if we were in the mood.

We definitely thought we had designed the epitome of classy after-school snacks. Fortunately, our palettes and cooking abilities have both evolved since then. These days, you won't often find me chowing down on a soggy microwave "quesadillas." You will, however, find me trying lots of healthy, grown-up recipes that pay homage to one of my earliest attempts in the kitchen.

This baked chicken quesadilla casserole is one of my favorite takes yet. Classic chicken quesadillas get a spicy twist with cumin and chili powder. Meanwhile, preparing this dish as a casserole makes for easy prep and a perfect weeknight meal.

- ✓ Yields: 8 servings

- ✓ Serving Size: 1 cup

- ✓ Calories: 354

- ✓ Total Fat: 13g

- ✓ Saturated Fat: 5g

- ✓ Trans Fat: 0g

- ✓ Cholesterol: 51mg

- ✓ Sodium: 533mg

- ✓ Carbohydrates: 35g

- ✓ Fiber: 6g

- ✓ Sugar: 1g

- ✓ Protein: 23g

- ✓ SmartPoints (Freestyle): 6

Ingredients

- ✓ 2 cups cooked and shredded chicken breast

- ✓ 1/2 cup (fat-free) sour cream

- ✓ 1 cup (reduced-fat) shredded cheddar cheese

- ✓ 2 teaspoons ground cumin

- ✓ 1 tablespoon chili powder

- ✓ 1 teaspoon Kosher salt

- ✓ 1/4 teaspoon ground black pepper

- ✓ 1 cup corn kernels (canned or frozen, thawed)

- ✓ 1 (15 ounce) can black beans, drained and rinsed

- ✓ 4 larger whole grain tortillas, recipe for tortillas

Instructions

- ✓ Preheat the oven o 400 degrees. Spray a 9 x 13 inch casserole dish with non stick spray.

- ✓ In a large bowl, combine the chicken, sour cream, half the cheese, half the cumin, half the chili powder, salt, and half the pepper. Mix well.

- ✓ In a second bowl, combine the corn, black beans, the remaining cumin, chili powder, and pepper. Mix well.

- ✓ Lay two of the tortillas in the bottom of the casserole dish. Spread half of the chicken mixture over the tortillas and half the bean mixture over the chicken. Place the remaining tortillas over the beans and repeat. Sprinkle the remaining cheese on top.

✓ Bake for 20 to 30 minutes or until cheese is melted. Serve hot.

Snack: Oven-Baked Zucchini Chips Smartpoints (Freestyle): 2

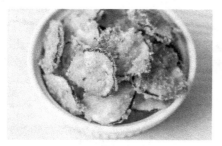

Move over potato chips – there's a new snack in town! Vending machine chips had a good run, but they're filled with saturated fat and other unpronounceable ingredients. Even though I know they're bad for me, I still reach for those processed chips all too often. They seemed to be the only thing that satisfies my urge for a crispy, crunchy snack. Luckily, we figured out a way for you to have your cake and eat it, too. These oven baked zucchini chips are low in fat and calories, and they're best described with one, simple word: yummy.

There's a good reason that zucchini is one of our favorite vegetables. It grows in abundance in the summertime and it's super easy to cook with. You can eat it raw as zoodles, sauté it as a stir-fry, slice it and toss it on the grill, or roast it in the oven. It's full of vitamins, minerals, and antioxidants. In fact, did you know that dark green zucchini boasts high levels of beta-carotene? That helps boost your immune system and promote healthy vision, too.

- ✓ Yields: 4 servings

- ✓ Calories: 99

- ✓ Total Fat: 3 g

- ✓ Saturated Fat: 2 g

- ✓ Trans Fat: 0 g

- ✓ Cholesterol: 13

- ✓ Carbohydrates: 12 g

- ✓ Sodium: 241 mg

- ✓ Dietary Fiber: 2 g

- ✓ Sugars: 2 g

- ✓ Protein: 6 g

- ✓ SmartPoints (Freestyle): 2 |

Ingredients

- ✓ 1 (large) zucchini, cut into 1/8" - 1/4" slices

- ✓ 1/3 cup whole grain breadcrumbs, optional Panko (homemade breadcrumb recipe)

✓ 1/4 cup finely grated parmesan cheese, reduced fat

✓ 1/4 teaspoon black pepper

✓ Kosher or sea salt to taste

✓ 1/8 teaspoon garlic powder

✓ 1/8 teaspoon cayenne pepper

✓ 3 tablespoons low-fat milk

Instructions

✓ Preheat oven to 425 degrees.

✓ Combine in a small mixing bowl, breadcrumbs, parmesan cheese, black pepper, salt, garlic powder, and cayenne pepper. Dip zucchini slices into milk and dredge into bread crumbs to coat both sides. Note: It may be necessary to press crumbs onto zucchini slices to ensure the crumbs stick.

✓ Arrange zucchini on a non-stick cookie sheet and lightly mist with a non-stick cooking spray.

✓ If using a rack, place rack on a cookie sheet. Bake 15 minutes, turn over and continue baking until golden, approximately 10-15 minutes (being careful not to burn). Allow to cool to room temperature before storing in an airtight container.

✓ TIP: Zucchini Chips will continue to get crispier while cooling.

✓ NOTE: For gluten free chips, use gluten-free bread crumbs.

DAY 4 (18 SMARTPOINTS)

Breakfast: Turkey Sausage Breakfast Muffins Smartpoints (Freestyle): 5

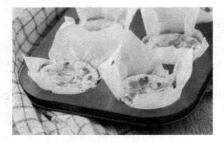

Busy schedules make it almost impossible to enjoy a quick, but nutritious breakfast. Which is why we love protein-packed, portable breakfast muffins! This Turkey Sausage Breakfast Muffin is not only packed with protein, but it will excite your tastebuds no matter how early in the morning. Who doesn't want to wake up to succulent turkey sausage chunks, crunchy bell peppers, and gooey cheese? The best part of this dish is that it can be prepared ahead of time so that it lasts the entire week. Plus, this make-ahead breakfast has the perfect balance of all the food groups. With just a little bit of everything, this recipe is all about the maximum **q**uality in minimum **q**uantity.

In order to whip up these savory snacks, all you have to do is sauté the veggies and meat, dice up the bread, and combine the rest of the ingredients, adding more or less of anything as you desire. In less than an hour, you can have up to 12 muffins ready to go. But beware, they may go fast!

✓ Yields: 12 muffins

✓ Serving Size: 1 muffin

✓ Calories: 162

✓ Total Fat: 9g

✓ Saturated Fat: 4g

✓ Trans Fat: 0g

✓ Cholesterol: 60mg

✓ Sodium: 332mg

✓ Carbohydrates: 7g

✓ Fiber: 1g

✓ Sugar: 1g

✓ Protein: 12g

✓ SmartPoints (Freestyle): 5

Ingredients

✓ 1/2 pound turkey sausage

✓ 1/4 cup green bell pepper, diced

✓ 1/4 cup red onion, diced

✓ 3 cups whole wheat bread, diced into 1/2 inch cubes

✓ 2 cup low fat shredded cheddar cheese

✓ 6 egg whites

✓ 2 eggs

✓ 1/4 cup skim milk

✓ 1/2 teaspoon Kosher salt

Instructions

✓ Preheat oven to 350 degrees. Line muffin tin with 12 paper muffin cup liners or lightly spray with non stick spray.

✓ In medium skillet, cook turkey sausage, breaking up into small pieces as it cooks. Cook until no pink remains. Add green pepper and onion to the sausage and cook until soft.

✓ Divide bread cubes between 12 muffin cups. Spoon turkey sausage mix on top of bread crumbs and cheese on top of the turkey mix. Only fill cups about 3/4 full.

✓ In a bowl, whisk together egg whites, eggs, milk, and salt. Pour over bread, sausage, and cheese filled muffin cups. Only fill to just cover the ingredients in the muffin cups. Allow to rest for 5 minutes and add more egg mix to the cups if needed.

✓ Bake for 15 to 20 minutes until set in the middle and tops begin to brown. Allow to rest for 5 minutes before removing from muffin tin. Serve warm.

Lunch: Mediterranean Chopped Salad With Salmon, Cucumber And Mint Smartpoints (Freestyle): 9

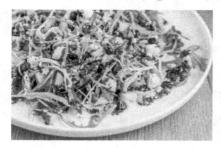

When summer rolls around, all I want to eat is salad. This is pretty convenient as far as my clean eating goals go, but that's not the only reason I'm drawn to salads. With an emphasis on light fare and fresh produce in abundance, summer just makes it so easy to eat healthy without even thinking about it.

While there is no shortage of salad recipes out there (as well as countless ways to mix things up off book), I often find myself falling into the same patterns when it comes to my salads. I'll find one flavor palette or combination of ingredients and just keep repeating it for days on end.

This Moroccan chicken salad with chimichurri dressing was a recent attempt to get out of a salad rut. And let me tell you, it worked. Moroccan food has such a unique, zesty flavor, and this salad captures it perfectly. This pretty salad bursts with fresh, tangy flavor that will definitely free you from any salad rut.

✓ Yields: 4 servings

✓ Serving Size: 1 1/2 cups salad, 2 tablespoons dressing

✓ Calories: 300 | Total Fat: 19g

✓ Saturated Fat:4g

✓ Trans Fat: 0g | Cholesterol: 70mg

✓ Sodium: 271mg

✓ Carbohydrates: 10g

✓ Fiber: 3g

✓ Sugar: 5g

✓ Protein: 23g

✓ SmartPoints (Freestyle): 6

Ingredients

For the Chimichurri Dressing:

✓ 1 clove garlic

✓ 1 cup fresh cilantro

✓ 1/4 cup fresh parsley

✓ 1 tablespoon lemon juice

✓ 3 tablespoons olive oil

✓ 1/4 teaspoon Kosher salt

✓ Pinch of crushed red pepper

For the Salad:

✓ 1 1/2 cups boneless and skinless chicken breast, cooked and shredded (leftovers work great)

✓ 6 cups baby arugula

✓ 1 cup shredded carrot

✓ 1 cup cucumber, chopped

✓ 1/4 cup pomegranate seeds

✓ 1/4 cup fat free feta cheese crumbles

✓ 1/4 cup chopped almonds

Instructions

For the Chimichurri Dressing:

✓ Combine all ingredients in a food processor and pulse until finely chopped and well mixed. Set aside

For the Salad:

✓ Combine all ingredients in a large bowl and toss. Divide into serving bowls and drizzle about 1 to 2 tablespoons of Chimichurri Dressing over top. Serve and enjoy.

Dinner: Clean Eating Pizza Lasagna Rolls Smartpoints (Freestyle): 7

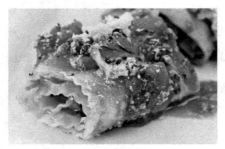

When you think of the most decadent of traditional Italian meals, what comes to mind? Some of us love the gooey, warm, creamy lasagna our grandmothers made. Others crave a hot slice of pizza, just out of the oven. You can enjoy pizza and lasagna in one single

bite with these delicious lasagna rolls, flavored with classic Italian pizza flavor, a combination of good *q*uality tomato sauce mixed with cheese, herbs, and extra virgin olive oil.

Make your own tomato sauce in minutes by combining sauteed garlic with tomato puree and oregano. Add three popular Italian cheeses, mozzarella, ricotta, and parmesan. Mozzarella gives a mild, mellow flavor and a gooey texture, ricotta adds the creamy texture, while Parmesan adds a salty bite that combines with tomato to create a classic flavor.

✓ Yields: 10 rolls

✓ 10 servings

✓ Serving Size: 1 roll

✓ Calories: 232

✓ Total Fat: 11 g

✓ Saturated Fat: 6 g

✓ Trayyyns Fat: 0 g

✓ Cholesterol: 25 mg

✓ Sodium: 573 mg

✓ Carbohydrates: 19 g

✓ Dietary Fiber: 3 g y

✓ Sugars: 1 g

✓ Protein: 14 g

✓ SmartPoints (Freestyle): 7

Ingredients

Sauce (optional: use 1 (24-ounce) jar marinara instead of homemade sauce)

✓ 2 cloves garlic, minced

✓ 1 tablespoon extra-virgin olive oil

✓ 2 (14-ounce) cans diced tomatoes with liquid

✓ 1 1/4 teaspoons dried oregano

✓ 1/2 teaspoon kosher or sea

✓ 1/4 teaspoon black pepper

Lasagna

✓ 1/2 cup parmesan cheese, grated

✓ 2 cups shredded part-skim mozzarella

✓ 1/2 cup ricotta cheese

✓ 1/4 teaspoon pepper

✓ 1 teaspoon dried oregano

✓ 10 whole grain lasagna noodles, boiled according to package

Instructions

✓ Over medium heat, in a saucepan with extra-virgin olive oil, sautè the garlic for 1 minute. Add the canned tomatoes, bring to a boil then lower the heat to a simmer. Season with salt, pepper, and dried oregano then simmer for 15 - 10 minutes.

✓ Preheat the oven to 375 degrees F.

✓ Pour 1 cup sauce in the bottom of a 13 x 9-inch casserole pan, set aside.

✓ Combine cheeses, pepper, and oregano. Evenly spread cheese mixture over each lasagna roll, retaining 1/2 cup for the top. Drizzle 1 tablespoon sauce over cheese. Roll to close, then place on the baking dish, seam side down.

✓ Pour 1 1/2 cups sauce over the top and sprinkle on remaining cheese mixture. Serve any remaining sauce with rolls. Loosely cover with foil and bake in the preheated oven for 25-30 minutes or until cheese is completely melted.

✓ Let the rolls rest for a few minutes before serving.

Snack: Baked Apple Chips SmartPoints (Freestyle): 0

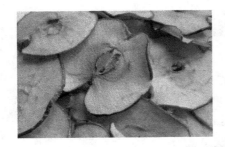

Previously, I wrote a short article. about the beginning of my weight loss journey. Fast forward a few months and here I am still losing weight. I thought it'd be extremely difficult and I never truly believed that I could keep the weight loss up. I started out at 240 pounds or more and now I weigh 169 pounds. I've even started a blog that documents my weight loss journey. I also post healthy recipes, talk about fashion, and other social issues. I hope you enjoy my recipe for Apple Chips.

- ✓ Yields: 6 servings

- ✓ Serving Size: 1/2 cup

- ✓ Calories: 32

- ✓ Total Fat: 0 g

- ✓ Saturated Fat: 0 g

- ✓ Trans Fat: 0 g

- ✓ Cholesterol: 0 mg

- ✓ Sodium: 1 mg

- ✓ Carbohydrates: 8.5 g

- ✓ Dietary Fiber: 1.6 g

- ✓ Sugars: 6.3 g

- ✓ Protein: 0 g

- ✓ SmartPoints: 0

Ingredients

- ✓ 2 apples, cored and thinly sliced

- ✓ Cinnamon to taste

Instructions

- ✓ Preheat oven to 275 degrees.

- ✓ Line a cookie sheet with parchment paper and place the pieces of sliced apple on top.

- ✓ Sprinkle with cinnamon (to taste).

- ✓ Bake at 275 degrees for two hours. After 60 minutes, turn them over so they bake evenly. You should check on them after 60 minutes and every 30 minutes after that because oven cook times vary and you don't want to burn them. Once they look nice and crispy remove them from the oven and allow to cool.

DAY 5 (17 SMARTPOINTS)

Breakfast: Souffle Omelette with Mushrooms SmartPoints (Freestyle): 1

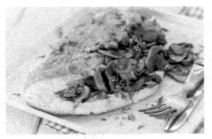

Imagine a big, hefty slice of a fluffy, soft omelette that's filled with sautèed mushrooms. Add in a touch of cheese and you'll have our healthy and delicious Soufflè Omelette with Mushrooms. It tastes so heavenly because we make it a bit differently from the normal omelette. Don't worry: We'll walk you through our super special (but, easy) method in a minute. You'll be an omelette-making pro in no time!

Omelettes are obviously a natural choice for breakfast because they're made with eggs. Don't be afraid to eat a dish like this Soufflè Omelette with Mushrooms for lunch or dinner, though. Being composed primarily of eggs, this dish is very rich in protein while being naturally low in carbs and sugar. Then you add in mushrooms, which are full of vitamins, minerals, and antioxidants. They also add a ton of flavor without adding much fat, calories, or cholesterol. The combination of both ingredients make this dish a powerhouse of nutrition!

✓ Yield: 6 servings

- ✓ Calories: 72

- ✓ Total Fat: 5 g

- ✓ Saturated Fat: 2 g

- ✓ Trans Fat: 0 g

- ✓ Carbohydrates: 2 g

- ✓ Fiber: 0 g

- ✓ Sugar: 1 g

- ✓ Protein: 6 g

- ✓ Cholesterol: 98 mg *-

- ✓ Sodium: 162 mg

- ✓ SmartPoints (Freestyle): 1

Ingredients

- ✓ 1 teaspoon extra-virgin olive oil

- ✓ 1 clove garlic, minced

- ✓ 8 ounces sliced mushrooms

- ✓ 1 tablespoon parsley, minced

- ✓ 3 large eggs, separated

✓ 1/2 teaspoon salt

✓ 1/2 teaspoon pepper

✓ 1/4 cup grated cheese

Instructions

✓ Over medium heat, in a skillet, warm olive oil and sautè the garlic.

✓ Add the mushrooms and sautè for 10 minutes. Add the parsley then turn off the heat. Set aside.

✓ Whisk the egg yolks, until thick. Next, beat the whites until white and frothy. (We used a blender for the egg whites). Fold the whites into the yolks, add cheese, and salt and pepper.

✓ Spray large skillet with nonstick spray.

✓ Pour in the egg mixture then cover. Cook until the top and bottom are set.

✓ With the help of a spatula, loosen it carefully. Add the mushrooms to the omelette then carefully fold over. Serve hot.

Lunch: Tuna Salad Stuffed Avocado SmartPoints (Freestyle): 8

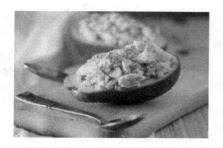

The combination of fresh tuna and avocado is a super punch of vitamins, minerals, and healthy fats! Our Tuna Salad Stuffed Avocado features a fresh seared tuna salad in an avocado bowl. The brightness of the lemon and Greek yogurt in the salad really balance the fattiness of the avocado to create a harmonious balance of flavors and textures.

This stuffed avocado makes for a refreshing and light lunch! It looks beautiful presented in the avocado halves, but you could certainly cut up the avocado and add it to the rest of the salad if you need to make it more portable.

✓ Yields: 2 servings

✓ Serving Size: 1/2 avocado/1/2 cup tuna salad

✓ Calories: 313

✓ Total Fat: 20g

✓ Saturated Fat: 3g

✓ Trans Fat: 0g

✓ Cholesterol: 36mg

✓ Sodium: 536mg

✓ Carbohydrates: 12g

✓ Fiber: 7g

✓ Sugar: 2g

✓ Protein: 25g

✓ SmartPoints (Freestyle): 8

Ingredients

✓ 1/2 tablespoon olive oil

✓ 6 ounce fresh tuna filet (such as ahi or blue fin tuna)

✓ 2 tablespoons plain Greek yogurt, optioal Clean Mayo

✓ 1 tablespoon lemon juice

✓ 2 tablespoons red onion, minced

✓ 1 tablespoon celery, minced

✓ 1/4 cup cucumber, diced small

✓ 1 teaspoon garlic powder

✓ 1/4 teaspoon cayenne pepper

✓ 1/2 teaspoon Kosher salt

✓ 1/2 teaspoon dry dill

✓ 1 whole avocado

Instructions

Heat olive oil in a skillet on medium heat. Once hot, add tuna filet and sear on each side to golden brown. Tuna should be firm and still slightly pink in the center. Remove from heat at cool.

✓ Once cool, diced tuna into small cube. Add remaining ingredients, except avocado, and lightly toss. Set aside.

OPTION: 2 (5 ounce) cans of tuna may be substituted for fresh tuna. Do not sear canned tuna, mix into other ingredients as directed. We recommend Safe Catch brand.

✓ Leaving peel on the avocado, cut in half, removing the pit. If needed carefully cut a "dent" into the center of each half to create a bowl.

✓ Divide tuna salad between each half, placing in the center of the avocado bowl. Serve and enjoy!

Dinner: Turkey Meatloaf Cupcakes with Mashed Potatoes SmartPoints (Freestyle): 6

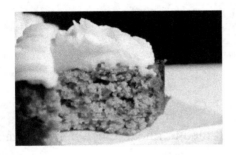

Nutritious cupcakes for dinner? You know it! Guaranteed fun for the whole family, this recipe stuffs muffin cups with a fluffy turkey meatloaf and tops each with mashed potato icing.

Our mouthwatering Turkey Meatloaf Cupcakes with Mashed Potatoes incorporate a delicious jumble of whole wheat bread crumbs, savory sauces, and flavorful herbs with lean, protein-packed turkey.

Unlike conventional mashed potato recipes, this one opts for lighter ingredients like low-fat milk. Pop the cupcakes in the fridge overnight and pack the satisfying delights for tomorrow's lunch.

✓ Yields: 6 servings

✓ Calories: 329

✓ Total Fat: 12g

✓ Saturated Fat: 3g

✓ Trans Fat: 0g

✓ Cholesterol: 120mg

- ✓ Sodium: 636mg

- ✓ Carbohydrates: 35g

- ✓ Fiber: 3g

- ✓ Sugar: 7g

- ✓ Protein: 22g

- ✓ SmartPoints (Freestyle): 6

Ingredients

- ✓ Meatloaf

- ✓ 1 pound lean ground turkey

- ✓ 1 egg, beaten

- ✓ 1/2 cup whole wheat breadcrumbs

- ✓ 1/4 cup ketchup

- ✓ 1/2 cup diced onion

- ✓ 1/2 cup grated carrots (grate on large holes of a cheese/box grater)

- ✓ 1/2 cup finely chopped fresh parsley leaves

- ✓ 1 clove garlic, minced, or 1 teaspoon garlic powder

✓ 2 teaspoons Worcestershire sauce

✓ 1/2 teaspoon kosher or sea salt

✓ 1/2 teaspoon black pepper

✓ 1 teaspoon dried oregano

✓ Mash

✓ 2 large russet potatoes, peeled and chopped

✓ 1 tablespoon extra virgin olive oil or butter

✓ 1/2 cup low-fat milk

✓ 1/4 teaspoon kosher or sea salt

Instructions

✓ Preheat oven to 350 degrees. Spray 12 cups of a muffin tin generously with cooking spray.

✓ Place potatoes in a pot of cold, salted water over high heat and bring to a boil. Reduce heat to medium-high. Cook until tender when pierced with a fork, about 20 minutes. Drain. Mash potatoes with olive oil, salt, and milk.

✓ Meanwhile, mix meatloaf ingredients in a large bowl. Hands may be used. Divide meatloaf evenly into 12 muffin cups, 3/4 of the way full, pressing the meat in.

✓ Bake for 35 minutes or until cooked through. The inside should read 165 degrees when pierced with a meat thermometer. Cool muffins for about 4 to 5 minutes, remove from tin, and spread each evenly with mashed potatoes, lifting spatula to create peaks if desired.

✓ Enjoy!

Snack: Southwestern Brussels Sprout Coleslaw SmartPoints (Freestyle): 2

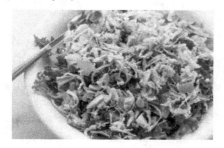

I have some pretty vivid memories of coleslaw. I know that might sound like a weird thing to remember from childhood, but it was such an iconic side at the neighborhood block party. No matter what the occasion -Memorial Day, Fourth of July, or Father's Day – a bowl of my mom's coleslaw was sure to make an appearance.

I still love her classic cabbage-mayonnaise-sugar slaw recipe. I make it all the time, but I've also been having a little bit of fun with coleslaw these days. The biggest eye-opener for me was a coleslaw I tasted that had Brussels sprouts as the main ingredient. I had no idea that you could make coleslaw without cabbage as the base! Now that I've tried this southwestern Brussels sprout cole-slaw, it totally makes sense, but it was mind-blowing the first time I tried it.

- ✓ Yields: 5 servings

- ✓ Serving Size: 1 cup

- ✓ Calories: 123

- ✓ Total Fat: 5g

- ✓ Saturated Fat: 1g

- ✓ Trans Fat: 0g

- ✓ Cholesterol: 0mg

- ✓ Sodium: 260mg

- ✓ Carbohydrates: 19g

- ✓ Fiber: 6g

- ✓ Sugar: 6g

- ✓ Protein: 4g

- ✓ SmartPoints (Freestyle): 2

Ingredients

- ✓ 4 cups Brussels sprouts, shaved or finely chopped

- ✓ 1 cup kale, roughly chopped

- ✓ 3 tablespoons red onion, finely minced

- ✓ 1/2 cup charred corn kernels

- ✓ 1 tablespoon jalapeno, minced

- ✓ 1/4 cup tomatoes, diced small

- ✓ 1/4 cup lime juice

- ✓ 1 cup avocado, mashed

- ✓ 2 teaspoons honey

- ✓ 1/2 teaspoon kosher salt

- ✓ 1 teaspoon ground cuming

- ✓ 1 table spoon chili powder

Instructions

- ✓ In a large mixing bowl, combine the Brussels sprouts, kale, corn, onion, jalapeno, and tomatoes. Lightly toss.

- ✓ In a small mixing bowl, combine the remaining ingredients to make a sauce. Add to the Brussels sprouts mixture and toss until everything is coated in the avocado sauce. Refrigerate for at least 30 minutes before serving. Enjoy!

DAY 6 (16 SMARTPOINTS)

Breakfast: Peanut Butter Banana Overnight Oats Smart-Points (Freestyle): 7

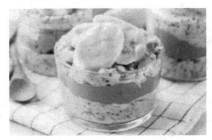

Peanut butter and banana are just one of those can't-lose combos. It's a tasty, hearty, and filling combination that creates a sweet treat that's also nutritionally rich. Peanut butter is famously high in protein. Meanwhile, bananas are a known powerhouse of nutrients, including high potassium and fiber levels. Together, these tasty ingredients make a hearty, instantly energizing meal. This Peanut Butter Banana Overnight Oats recipe is certainly no exception.

With all the delicious, energizing health benefits of peanut butter and bananas, this quick and easy make-ahead breakfast recipe will definitely satisfy. It also boosts its nutritional profile with almond milk and chia seeds. It's the perfect sweet and tasty, high-protein way to start your day.

✓ Yield: about 2 cups

✓ Servings: 2 servings

✓ Calories: 227

✓ Total Fat: 11 g

✓ Saturated Fat: 2 g

✓ Trans Fat: 0 g

✓ Carbohydrates: 40 g

✓ Fiber: 5 g

✓ Sugar: 9 g

✓ Protein: 7 g

✓ Cholesterol: 0 mg

✓ Sodium: 47 mg

✓ SmartPoints (Freestyle): 7

Ingredients

✓ 1/2 cup rolled oats

✓ 1 cup almond milk

✓ 1 tablespoon chia seeds

✓ 1/4 teaspoon vanilla extract

✓ 1/2 teaspoon ground cinnamon

✓ 1 tablespoon honey, (maple syrup for a vegan option)

✓ 1 banana, sliced

✓ 2 tablespoons natural creamy peanut butter

Instructions

✓ Combine the oats, milk, chila seeds, vanilla, cinnamon, and honey. Mix well. Pour a small amount into 2 glass jars or other serving containers.

✓ Layer the banana and peanut butter and pour the remaining oat mixture over top. Cover, seal, and let sit overnight. Serve chilled.

Lunch: Tomato, Mozzarella, and Basil Panini SmartPoints (Freestyle): 8

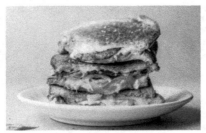

I'm all about grilled cheese! There's something so satisfying about the way that crispy bread combines with melted cheese. When I was a kid, there's no way I would eat anything other than white bread and cheddar cheese. Today, I'm happy to report that my picky-eating tendencies didn't extend into my adulthood! Tomato, mozzarella, and basil are mouthwatering members of classic Italian combinations, and you usually see them in caprese salads. You'll be thrilled to learn that we've combined these ingredients with a classic grilled cheese to create a savory Tomato Mozzarella and Basil Panini.

This sandwich has so much going on! Whole wheat bread slices, juicy tomatoes, spicy red onions, fresh basil, mozzarella cheese, and heart-healthy olive oil; what more could you ask for? Using a panini press (or a regular old skillet), we cook the sandwich, flattening it out as much as possible, to create golden-brown, super crispy bread. Inside, you'll find tomatoes bursting with sweet and savory flavor and creamy, melted cheese that pairs perfectly with the bold flavors of the basil. It's kind of perfect!

- ✓ Yields: 2 servings

- ✓ Serving Size: 1/2 sandwich

- ✓ Calories: 231

- ✓ Total Fat: 13g

- ✓ Saturated Fat: 6g

- ✓ Trans Fat: 0g

- ✓ Cholesterol: 25mg

- ✓ Sodium: 475mg

✓ Carbohydrates: 15g

✓ Fiber: 2g

✓ Sugar: 3g

✓ Protein: 10g

✓ SmartPoints (Freestyle): 8

Ingredients

✓ 2 slices whole wheat bread

✓ 1/2 cup shredded part-skim mozzarella

✓ 1 Roma tomato, thinly sliced

✓ 1 thin slice of red onion

✓ 8 fresh basil leaves

✓ Pinch of kosher or sea salt

✓ 1/8 teaspoon pepper

✓ 1 tablespoon extra-virgin olive oil

Instructions

✓ Spread olive oil with a pastry or basting brush over two slices of bread. Sprinkle each with salt and pepper.

✓ Place one of the bread slices, oil-side down and top basil leaves, tomato slices, onion, and mozzarella. Top with other piece of bread, olive oil side up.

✓ Place a heavy-bottomed skillet on the stovetop over medium-high heat or use a Panini press.

✓ If using a skillet, press down with lid to flatten sandwich a bit. Cook for about 2 minutes, until golden on the bottom, and flip. Repeat on other side.

✓ Slice sandwich in half to make 2 servings.

✓ Enjoy!

Dinner: Slow Cooker Balsamic Chicken SmartPoints (Freestyle): 1

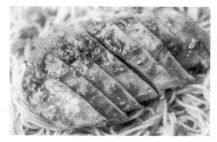

We love Italian cuisine., but we're not always in the mood for heavy pastas and sauces. When we're looking to serve something a little lighter for dinner, but we don't want to sacrifice the zesty Italian flavor we've come to love, this Slow Cooker Balsamic Chicken does the trick! This slow cooker recipe is easy to make, healthy, and tastes delicious. Chicken recipes do not have to be boring. Slow cooker foods are a great way to pack a lot of flavor into lean chicken breast. The end result of this balsamic chicken recipe is a moist, flavorful dish your entire family will love!

✓ Yields: 10 Cups

✓   Serving size: 1 Cup

✓ Calories: 238

✓ Fat: 12 g

✓   Saturated fat: 3 g

✓ Trans fat: 0 g

✓   Cholesterol: 73 mg

✓   Sodium: 170 mg

✓ Carbohydrate: 7 g

✓   Fiber: 2 g

✓   Sugar: 4 g

✓   Protein 25 g

✓   Smart Points (Freestyle): 1

Ingredients

- ✓ 4-6 boneless, skinless, chicken breasts (about 40 ounces)

- ✓ 2 14.5 oz can diced tomatoes

- ✓ 1 medium onion thinly sliced (Not chopped)

- ✓ 4 garlic cloves

- ✓ 1/2 cup balsamic vinegar (for gluten-free use White Balsamic Vinegar which doesn't have caramel coloring)

- ✓ 1 tablespoon olive oil

- ✓ 1 teaspoon dried oregano

- ✓ 1 teaspoon dried basil

- ✓ 1 teaspoon dried rosemary

- ✓ 1/2 teaspoon thyme

- ✓ ground black pepper and salt to taste

Instructions

- ✓ Pour the olive oil on bottom of slow cooker, add chicken breasts, salt and pepper each breast, put sliced onion on top of chicken then put in all the dried herbs and garlic cloves. Pour in vinegar and top with tomatoes.

- ✓ Cook on high 4 hours, serve over angel hair pasta.

Snack: Instant Pot Applesauce SmartPoints (Freestyle): 0

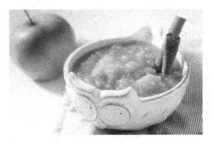

If you're running out of ideas of what snacks to give your kids, you've come to the right place. This recipe will become your favorite as well as theirs! Everyone loves a good applesauce, but how often do we actually try our hand at making it? There's always a first time, and for your first attempt you'll love this fail-safe Instant Pot applesauce. With 4 ingredients and 20 minutes, you can accomplish nearly perfect applesauce that your kids will fall in love with. You simply need the Instant Pot in order to cook the apples and soak in the cinnamon and lime juice. Once the apples have cooked, they go straight into a blender and come out as the final product. It's so easy to do and just as easy to eat. Give it a go, and see how many servings your kids ask for!

✓ Yields: 4 servings

✓ Calories: 177

✓ Total Fat: 1g

✓ Saturated Fat: 0g

✓ Trans Fat: 0g

✓ Cholesterol: 0mg

✓ Sodium: 5mg

✓ Carbohydrates: 42g

✓ Fiber: 9g

✓ Sugar: 22g

✓ Protein: 1g

✓ SmartPoints (Freestyle): 0

Ingredients

✓ 6 to 8 medium apples (we recommend a combination of Granny Smith and Gala apples

✓ 1 cup water

✓ 1 teaspoon lemon juice

2 teaspoons cinnamon (optional)

Instructions

✓ Peel and cut apples into 2 inch chunks. Place apples and all other ingredients into the Instant Pot.

✓ Close Instant Pot lid,ensuring the vent is in the sealed position. Press the "manual" button and adjust to high pressure and set the timer to 8 minutes. The Instant Pot will preheat before beginning the cooking time.

✓ Once the timer goes off, let sit for about 2-3 minutes. Turn steam vent to release pressure and carefully release the steam and remove lid.

✓ Drain off any excess water. Place cooked apples in a mixture and mix on low until desired applesauce consistency is reached - smooth or chunky! Allow to cool slightly before serving.

✓ NOTE: This recipe can also be used when canning or freezing applesauce!

DAY 7 (21 SMARTPOINTS)

Breakfast: Peanut Butter Mocha Espresso Shake Smartpoints (Freestyle): 11

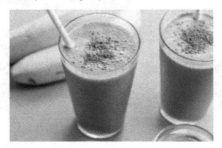

There are a ton of classic combinations out there: ham and cheese, milk and cookies, or apples and cinnamon. These combinations work because the flavors complement each other so well, they make our taste buds do a happy dance! One of my favorite combinations has to be peanut butter and chocolate. Salty, savory peanut butter alongside rich and creamy chocolate simply makes my palate sing. The most iconic example of this is a Reeses candy bar, but that's not exactly the best use of my calories! When I'm craving a sweet treat, I've started turning to this Peanut Butter Mocha Espresso Shake.It satisfies all my sweet tooth cravings without filling me up with empty calories.

You'll get protein from the peanut butter, calcium from the almond milk, and potassium and fiber from the naturally sweet banana. And, since we threw some coffee into the mix, you'll also get a burst of caffeine-fueled energy. Talk about a perfect way to start your day!

✓ Yield: 1 Serving

✓ Serving Size: 1 Shake

✓ Calories: 179

✓ Total Fat: 10 g

✓ Saturated Fat: 3 g

✓ Trans Fat: 0 g

✓ Carbohydrates: 21 g

✓ Fiber: 6 g

✓ Sugar: 9 g

✓ Protein: 6 g

✓ Cholesterol: 0 mg

✓ Sodium: 97 mg

✓ SmartPoints (Freestyle): 7

Ingredients

✓ 1/2 frozen banana

✓ 1 tablespoon peanut butter

✓ 1 tablespoon unsweetened cocoa powder

✓ 1/2 cup almond milk

✓ 1/2 cup strong brewed coffee, chilled

✓ 3/4 cup ice

Instructions

✓ Combine all ingredients in a blender. Blend until smooth.

Lunch: Skinny Taco Salad in a Jar SmartPoints (Freestyle): 3

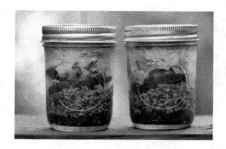

While many taco salad recipes are topped with full fat cheese, rich sour cream, and fried tortillas, our version is full of southwest flavor, made with wholesome, clean ingredients like ground turkey and fresh tomatoes. Layer these in a jar with an easy homemade salsa avocado dressing for a *q*uick taco salad in a jar that you can take with you to work, or store in the fridge for an *q*uick meal.

✓ *includes the dressing Yields: 6 servings

✓ Serving Size: 1-1/4 cup (fits well in a pint-sized jar)

✓ Calories: 196

✓ Total Fat: 12 g

✓ Saturated Fat: 5 g

✓ Trans Fat: 0 g

✓ Cholesterol: 48 mg

✓ Sodium: 469 mg

✓ Carbohydrates: 9 g

✓ Dietary Fiber: 2 g

✓ Sugars: 3 g

✓ Protein: 15 g

✓ SmartPoints (Freestyle): 3

Ingredients

Salad:

✓ 1/2 pound ground turkey

✓ 1 teaspoon chili powder

✓ 1/2 teaspoon cumin

✓ 1/4 teaspoon garlic powder

✓ 1/4 teaspoon sea salt

✓ 1/2 cup whole grain tortilla chips, broken

✓ 1/2 cup shredded cheddar cheese, reduced-fat

✓ 3 cups chopped romaine lettuce

✓ 1 cup halved cherry tomatoes

✓ 1/2 cup salsa, no sugar added

✓ Creamy Salsa Dressing: (optional)

✓ 2 tablespoons plain Greek yogurt

✓ 2 tablespoons ripe, mashed avocado

✓ Juice of 1 lime

✓ 1/4 cup salsa

Instructions

✓ Heat a skillet over medium heat and add the turkey. Cook until turkey is no longer pink and cooked through. Add spices, stir to combine and transfer to a bowl and let cool.

✓ To make the salad, divide the tortilla chips between six jars. Layer each with the salsa, turkey mixture, tomatoes, lettuce, and cheese.

✓ Make the optional dressing by blending the yogurt, avocado, lime juice, and salsa in a blender. Blend until creamy and smooth. Top the salad with the dressing, seal the jars and store in the fridge until ready to eat. Eat within 1-2 days for best results.

Dinner: Skinny Zucchini Pasta & Baby Spinach Smart-Points (Freestyle): 4

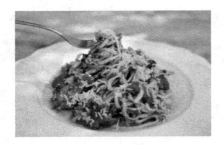

When warm weather comes knockin' and vegetable season rolls around, whip up some Skinny Zucchini Pasta & Baby Spinach!

Flavorful and tasty, especially in season, zucchini tops the charts in terms of powerful superfoods. The veggie does so much more than offer a host of health benefits. It's super versatile, starring in countless dishes in a variety of roles. Fresh zucchini disguised as pasta noodles pairs beautifully with baby spinach in this healthy recipe.

This light, satisfying dish is bursting with essential nutrients. Topped with a mouthwatering medley of garlic, olive oil, tomatoes, and savory spices, the two superfoods soak up amazing flavor. Sprinkle some parmesan on top for a fabulous finish, and voila! This recipe will have the kids gobbling up their veggies without hesitation.

- ✓ Yields: 6 servings

- ✓ Calories: 116

- ✓ Total Fat: 8g

- ✓ Saturated Fat: 2g

✓ Trans Fat: 0g

✓ Cholesterol: 6mg

✓ Sodium: 505mg

✓ Carbohydrates: 8g

✓ Fiber: 3g

✓ Sugar: 5g

✓ Protein: 6g

✓ SmartPoints (Freestyle): 4

Ingredients

✓ 4 medium zucchini, peeled and ends removed

✓ 1 teaspoon kosher or sea salt

✓ 2 tablespoons extra-virgin olive oil

✓ 3 cloves garlic, minced

✓ 1 (15 ounce) can diced tomatoes

✓ 1 tablespoon capers

✓ 1/4 cup Italian parsley

✓ 1 1/2 teaspoons dried oregano

✓ 1/2 teaspoon black pepper

✓ 1/4 teaspoon crushed red pepper flakes

✓ 1 cup loosely packed baby spinach

✓ 1/2 cup freshly grated parmesan cheese

Instructions

✓ Place each zucchini on a vegetable spiralizer to make the pasta. Use the smaller holes for spaghetti.

✓ Optional: Sprinkle 1/2 teaspoon salt on zucchini pasta, tossing to coat. Spread pasta on double layer of paper towels on a baking sheet, which will extract some of the water. Allow to set for 10 minutes.

✓ Add olive oil to a large skillet over medium-low heat.

✓ Add garlic and sauté for 1 minute.

✓ Raise heat to medium, add tomatoes with liquid, capers, parsley, oregano, black pepper, red pepper, remaining salt, and zucchini pasta, tossing to combine.

✓ Cook until pasta is tender, about 7-8 minutes.

✓ Add spinach and cook just until wilted, about 1 minute.

✓ Add to serving platter and sprinkle with parmesan.

✓ Enjoy!

Snack: Baked Onion Rings SmartPoints (Freestyle): 3

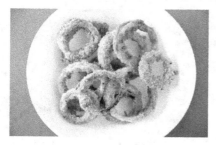

Need a little more crunch in your life? And maybe a little more flavor? And maybe something like fried food, but without all the guilt? Introducing SkinnyMs. baked onion rings! In their words, "We are onion rings with all the satisfying crunch and all the fun flavor -but without the fried fat. We're baked!"

Nothing says summertime like some good old fashioned onion rings. They're great for parties, great for snacks, and great for kiddie finger food. And they're easy to make -you only need an onion, some bread crumbs, flour, baking powder, an egg, salt & pepper, and milk -and you're good to bake! After just 20 painless minutes (ok, they might be a little bit painful because of the anticipation . . .), you will have an enviable treat to share -or not! Hey, no judgment here.

Add these crunchy baked onion rings to your favorite casseroles or have as an appetizer. Either way, they are delicious!

✓ Yields: 4 servings

✓ Serving Size: 1/4 of recipe

✓ Calories: 111

✓ Total Fat: 1 g

✓ Saturated Fat: 0 g

✓ Trans Fat: 0 g

✓ Cholesterol: 3

✓ Carbohydrates: 15 g

✓ Sodium: 139 mg

✓ Dietary Fiber: 2 g

✓ Sugars: 5 g

✓ Protein: 11 g

✓ SmartPoints (Freestyle): 3

Ingredients

✓ 1 large sweet or red onion, thinly sliced into rings

✓ 1/2 cup gluten-free Panko, or whole grain bread crumbs (bread crumb recipe)

- ✓ 1/2 cup flour, optional gluten free flour

- ✓ 1/2 teaspoon baking power

- ✓ 1/4 teaspoon black pepper

- ✓ Kosher or sea salt to taste

- ✓ 1 egg white

- ✓ 3/4 cup low-fat milk or low-fat buttermilk

Instructions

- ✓ Preheat oven to 400 degrees.

- ✓ In a medium mixing, combine panko or whole wheat bread crumbs, flour, salt, pepper and baking powder. Separate the onion slices into individual rings and add to the flour mixture, gently toss and make sure all the rings are coated. Remove onions and set aside.

- ✓ Whisk together milk and egg white, add to the leftover flour mixture and stir to combine. Dip onion rings into batter, allow excess to drip off and place on a non-stick cookie sheet. Lightly spray or drizzle extra-virgin olive oil on the onion rings. Flip onion rings after 10 minutes. Continue baking until golden and crispy, 10 to 15 additional minutes.

✓ Note: If using this recipe for Green Bean Casserole, reduce cooking time by 5 minutes as the onion rings will continue to brown while on top of the casserole.

DAY 8 (16 SMARTPOINTS)

Breakfast: Rise and Shine With These Greek Egg Muffins SmartPoints (Freestyle): 1

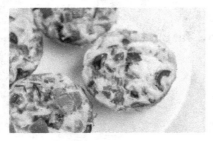

For those of us who are all about eggs for breakfast, it can be tough to find good on-the-go breakfast options. Fortunately, this Greek egg muffin recipe is about to change that.

Plenty of egg dishes are easy enough to whip up on busy mornings. But when you need something you can grab on your way to the car, a plate of scrambled eggs just isn't going to cut it.

Egg sandwiches are an easy enough solution, but not ideal for the carb-conscious. A good old-fashioned hard boiled egg will do the trick, but it's a pretty bland way to start your day.

If you're looking for an easy way to enjoy a warm egg breakfast on the go, this Greek egg muffin recipe is your new go to. Just a few fresh ingredients and a muffin tin are all you need for a super easy, grab-and-go breakfast.

To enjoy these egg muffins on busy mornings all week long, just make ahead, refrigerate, and reheat. Instead of grabbing another granola bar on your way out, you can actually have a hot egg breakfast. Just pop an egg muffin in the microwave on a busy morning and start your day with a protein packed, low carb breakfast on the go.

- ✓ Yields: 6 servings

- ✓ Serving Size: 1 egg muffin

- ✓ Calories: 45

- ✓ Total Fat: 2g

- ✓ Saturated Fat: 1g

- ✓ Trans Fat: 0g

- ✓ Cholesterol: 54mg

- ✓ Sodium: 155mg

- ✓ Carbohydrates: 2g

- ✓ Fiber: 0g

- ✓ Sugar: 2g

- ✓ Protein: 5g

- ✓ SmartPoints (Freestyle): 1

Ingredients

- ✓ 2 eggs

- ✓ 4 egg whites

- ✓ 1/2 cup skim milk

- ✓ 1/2 teaspoon Kosher salt

- ✓ 1/4 teaspoon ground white pepper

- ✓ 1/4 cup tomatoes, diced small

- ✓ 1/4 cup red onion, diced small

- ✓ 1/4 cup black olives, diced small

- ✓ 1 tablespoon fresh parsley, roughly chopped

- ✓ 1/4 cup fat free feta cheese, crumbled, (optional)

Instructions

- ✓ Preheat oven to 350 and spray a 6 count muffin tin with non-stick spray.

- ✓ In a mixing bowl, combine the eggs, milk, salt and pepper. Whisk well until slightly frothy. Stir in remaining ingredients.

- ✓ Fill muffin tin with the egg mixture, filling each muffin cup about 3/4 full. Bake for 15-20 minutes or until the egg muffins have cooked through and lightly browned on top. Serve immediately or store and reheat for a **q**uick grab and go breakfast!

Lunch: Clean Eating Chicken Salad Smartpoints (Freestyle): 2

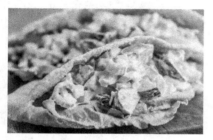

I'm sure we've all had more than a few versions of chicken salad. So many of them are mayonnaise-laden and heavy, filling us up with more unhealthy fats than we need. It shouldn't have to be that way, though. This dish has so much potential – it's a convenient topping for a healthy lunch or dinner, and it's a protein-packed powerhouse. So, we came up with a clean eating chicken salad recipe that will nourish your body and please your palate.

It's not just about tasting great and feeling light, either. Our clean eating chicken salad recipe is super easy to make and works well for meal prepping options for weekday lunches. Or, you can eat it on the weekend in the great outdoors as a picnic! Your whole family will love it, especially when they learn how this recipe goes one step further in helping you meet your weight loss goals.

✓ Servings: 4

✓ Calories: 291

✓ Total Fat: 11 g

✓ Saturated Fat: 4 g

✓ Trans Fat: 0 g

✓ Cholesterol: 60 mg

✓ Sodium: 486 mg

✓ Carbohydrates: 25 g

✓ Dietary Fiber: 3 g

✓ Sugars: 5 g

✓ Protein: 25 g

✓ SmartPoints: 2

Ingredients

2 cooked skinless, boneless chicken breasts - cut into cubes

✓ 2 celery stalks, chopped

✓ 1/4 red onion, chopped

✓ 1/2 cup red seedless grapes, quartered

✓ 1/2 cup Greek yogurt, non-fat

- ✓ 1 tsp garlic powder

- ✓ 1 tsp freshly ground black pepper

- ✓ Sea salt to taste

- ✓ 2 whole-wheat pita pockets, halved

- ✓ 4 romaine lettuce leaves

Instructions

- ✓ In a large bowl, mix all of the salad ingredients. Chicken salad can be eaten as is or eat as a pita sandwich. Recipe serves 4.

Dinner: 6-Ingredient Mexican Style Quinoa Salad Smartpoints (Freestyle): 5

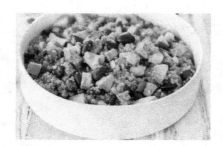

Quinoa can make any salad extra special with the nutrients it imparts. Considered one of nature's best superfoods, it's packed with vitamins and minerals that are essential for our health. It's rich in heart-healthy monounsaturated fats, omega-3 fatty acids, manganese, vitamin E, and many other wonderful nutrients. This

6-Ingredient Mexican-Style Quinoa Salad contains an incredible mixture of flavors. Zesty tomato salsa, fiber- and protein-rich black beans, and superfood avocado burst with flavor and amp up the salad's nutritional value. Add a can of corn to make this nutritious salad filled with colors, flavors, and nutrients pop. Dish up and enjoy!

- ✓ Yields: 4 servings

- ✓ Serving Size: about 3/4 cup

- ✓ Calories: 323

- ✓ Total Fat: 10 g

- ✓ Saturated Fat: 1 g

- ✓ Trans Fat: 0 g

- ✓ Cholesterol: 0 mg

- ✓ Sodium: 630 mg

- ✓ Carbohydrates: 49 g

- ✓ Fiber: 15 g

- ✓ Sugar: 4 g

- ✓ Protein: 13 g

- ✓ SmartPoints (Freestyle): 5

Ingredients

- ✓ 1/2 cup dry *q*uinoa, pre-rinsed

- ✓ 1 (15-ounce) can black beans, drained and rinsed

- ✓ 1 cups salsa, no-sugar added

- ✓ 1 cup corn kernels

- ✓ 1 teaspoon chili powder

- ✓ 1 avocado, peeled and small diced

Instructions

- ✓ Add 1 cup water and *q*uinoa to a medium pot and bring to a rolling boil over medium-high heat. Reduce heat to a simmer, cover and cook until most moisture is absorbed, about 12-15 minutes. Turn off heat and leave covered quinoa on burner for 5 minutes.

- ✓ Add to cooked quinoa, black beans, salsa, corn, and chili powder. Add salt and pepper to taste. Toss to combine then add diced avocado and gently toss. Add salad to a serving dish and serve. Salad can also be enjoyed cold.

- ✓ Enjoy!

Snack: Coconut Banana Paleo Cookies Smartpoints (Freestyle): 8

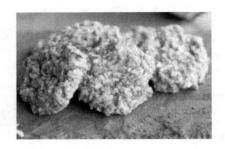

Channel your inner caveman with these scrumptious coconut banana paleo cookies! Our stone-aged ancestors probably weren't feasting on these tasty treats. However, this paleo-friendly recipe calls for nothing but 100% wholesome ingredients, all of which prehistoric people would've had access to.

Forget conventional cookie ingredients like white flour, butter, and refined sugar. This recipe opts for cleaner, healthier substitutes like almond meal and coconut oil to give the baked goods their delectably chewy texture and touch of sweetness.

Don't toss out those squishy bananas sitting on your counter collecting brown spots! Overripe bananas lend moist and flavorful character to each cookie that pairs perfectly with scrumptious shredded coconut. Perfect for satisfying any sweet tooth, these paleo-friendly delights let you enjoy cookies guilt-free!

✓ Yields: 18 servings

✓ Serving Size: 1 cookie

✓ Calories: 194

✓ Total Fat: 15g

- ✓ Saturated Fat: 5g

- ✓ Trans Fat: 0g

- ✓ Cholesterol: 17mg

- ✓ Sodium: 148mg

- ✓ Carbohydrates: 13g

- ✓ Fiber: 3g

- ✓ Sugar: 9g

- ✓ Protein: 5g

- ✓ SmartPoints (Freestyle): 8

Ingredients

- ✓ 3 cups almond flour

- ✓ 1 teaspoon baking soda

- ✓ 1/2 teaspoon kosher or sea salt

- ✓ 1 teaspoon cinnamon

- ✓ 1/4 cup (grass-fed) unsalted butter, room temperature, (optional coconut oil)

- ✓ 3/4 cup coconut sugar

- ✓ 1 large egg, beaten

- ✓ 1 large egg white

- ✓ 1 teaspoon pure vanilla

- ✓ 1 overly ripe banana (1/2 cup), mashed

- ✓ 1 cup finely shredded coconut, unsweetened

- ✓ 1 cup walnut pieces

Instructions

- ✓ Whisk together in a medium bowl, almond flour, baking soda, salt, and cinnamon. Add walnuts and coconut, and stir into flour mixture.

- ✓ In a medium mixing bowl, using a beater, cream together butter and coconut sugar. Add egg, egg white, and vanilla, mixing until combined. Stir in mashed banana and coconut, until combined.

- ✓ Add flour mixture to wet ingredients and stir just until incorporated. Cover and refrigerate 45 minutes.

- ✓ Preheat oven to 350 degrees.

- ✓ Using an 1-1/2 inch cookie or ice cream scoop, drop dough 2-inches apart on a large, parchment lined, cookie sheet. Bake 8 minutes and rotate cookie sheet. Bake an additional

8 minutes, or until golden and just set. Allow cookies to cool 5 minutes while still on the cookie sheet. Move cookies to a wire rack and cool completely. Continue baking cookies until all dough is used.

✓ Store in an airtight container up to two days. If desired, add 1 cup Paleo friendly chocolate chips when adding the walnuts.

DAY 9 (11 SMARTPOINTS)

Breakfast: Crustless Vegetable Quiche Smartpoints (Freestyle): 2

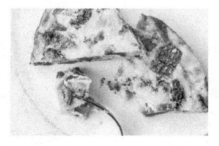

Eggs are a fantastic option for breakfast or brunch because they are such a terrific source of protein. Unfortunately, finding creative ways to prepare eggs can be a challenge. Quiche is a great option for adding variety and flavor to your morning serving of eggs, but the crust can be loaded with saturated fat and calories. Luckily, it is possible to enjoy a crustless vegetable quiche recipe that tastes great without the excess fat!

The other thing I love about this crustless vegetable **q**uiche is how easy it is to make. You don't have to worry about pre-baking the crust because there isn't any. All it takes is about 15 minutes of prep. Then, you just pour the egg mixture over the vegetables and bake it until it's golden brown and delicious. It doesn't get easier than that! That makes this a no-fuss way to cook eggs, and it's also a great way to feed a crowd, too.

- ✓ Yields: 6 servings

- ✓ serving size: 1 slice

- ✓ Calories: 141

- ✓ ü Total Fat: 5 g

- ✓ Saturated Fats: 1 g

- ✓ Trans Fats: 0 g

- ✓ Cholesterol: 93 mg

- ✓ Sodium: 593 mg

- ✓ Carbohydrates: 15 g

- ✓ Dietary fiber: 5 g

- ✓ Sugars: 5 g

- ✓ Protein: 11 g

✓ SmartPoints (Freestyle): 2

Ingredients

✓ 1 tablespoon olive oil

✓ 1 small yellow onion, diced

✓ 2 cloves garlic, mined

✓ ½ cup diced red bell pepper

✓ ½ cup diced green bell pepper

✓ ½ cup sliced zucchini

✓ 6 broccoli florets

✓ ¼ cup diced sun-dried tomatoes

✓ 3 large eggs

✓ 4 large egg whites

✓ 2 tablespoons low-fat milk

✓ 1 teaspoon dried oregano

✓ ½ teaspoon black pepper

✓ Sea Salt to taste

✓ ¼ cup plus 1 tablespoon low-fat parmesan cheese, optional

Instructions

✓ Preheat oven to 425 degrees.

✓ In a large skillet on medium-low heat, add oil and sauté onion and garlic until tender, about 4 minutes. Add diced bell pepper, zucchini, broccoli and sun-dried tomatoes and continue sautéing 2 minutes.

✓ In a medium mixing bowl, whisk together eggs, egg whites, milk, spices and ¼ cup parmesan cheese. Lightly spray a 9" pie dish, add sautéed vegetables. Pour egg mixture over vegetables, make sure to cover all veggies.

✓ Loosely cover with foil and bake 10 minutes at 425 degrees, reduce heat to 350 and continue baking 20-25 minutes. Remove foil the last few minutes of baking time and sprinkle with the remaining parmesan cheese. Quiche is done when it puffs and a knife inserted in the center comes out clean.

Lunch: Tomato, Hummus, And Spinach Sandwich Smartpoints (Freestyle): 3

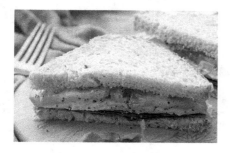

If you long for the days when you could just slap together a simple sandwich and call lunch done, we've got great news for you. This fresh and *q*uick Tomato, Hummus, and Spinach sandwich is easier to make than sliced bread.

Savory storebought hummus (pick your favorite flavor!) adds quick flavor and oodles of plant-based protein to your afternoon. The addition of a bright, ripe tomato and crunchy lettuce or spinach leaves makes for a perfect flavor match (with superfood benefits).

Hungry for a lunch that satisfies? Grab a loaf of your favorite mulitgrain or gluten-free bread, and prep this sandwich. You'll be enjoying a healthful meal in just 60 seconds or less. You body (and tastebuds) will thank you for it!

- ✓ Yields: 2 servings

- ✓ Serving Size: 1/2 sandwich

- ✓ Calories: 100

- ✓ Total Fat: 3 g

✓ Saturated Fat: 0 g

✓ Trans Fat: 0 g

✓ Cholesterol: 0 mg

✓ Sodium: 308 mg

✓ Carbohydrates: 15 g

✓ Dietary Fiber: 3 g

✓ Sugars: 2 g

✓ Protein: 5 g

✓ SmartPoints (Freestyle): 3

Ingredients

✓ 2 slices multigrain bread

✓ 2 tablespoons roasted garlic hummus, or hummus of choice

✓ 3 slices tomato

✓ 1/2 cup baby spinach

✓ 1/8 teaspoon salt (a pinch sprinkled on)

✓ Instructions

✓ Toast multigrain bread (if desired). Spread hummus on top of one slice of bread. Top with tomato slices and layer with spinach. Spinkle on salt. Place the second slice of bread on top. Serve and enjoy!

Dinner: Slow Cooker Spinach Artichoke Chicken Smart-points (Freestyle): 5

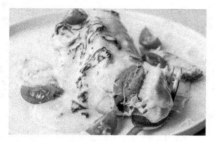

If you like the popular appetizer dip, you're going to go crazy over this recipe! Our Slow Cooker Spinach Artichoke Chicken takes all the flavor from the dip and turns it into a delicious dinner. It's still as tender and creamy as the delicious appetizer, but with a fraction of the calories. Not only that but since we cooked it up with chicken, you won't need to waste your carbs on dipping bread!

This simple, slow cooker chicken recipe looks gourmet, but it's so easy to make. You just toss the ingredients into the Crock Pot and turn it on low for six to eight hours. The chicken will be melt-in-your-mouth tender, and that sauce is so creamy, you won't believe it's actually healthy! This recipe is perfect for lazy autumn weekends or wowing company at a dinner party.

✓ Yields: 4 servings

✓ Serving Size: 1 chicken breast and 1/4 of the spinach, tomatoes, and artichokes

✓ Calories: 246

✓ Total Fat: 6 g

✓ Saturated Fat: 2 g

✓ Trans Fat: 0 g

✓ Cholesterol: 82 mg

✓ Sodium: 243 mg

✓ Carbohydrates: 14 g

✓ Dietary Fiber: 4 g

✓ Sugars: 3 g

✓ Protein: 35 g

✓ SmartPoints (Freestyle): 5

Ingredients

✓ 8 cups loosely packed spinach, chopped

✓ 1 cup chicken broth

- ✓ 4 (6-8 ounce) whole chicken breasts (bone-in with skin)

- ✓ 3 cloves fresh garlic, chopped

- ✓ 1/4 sweet onion, finely chopped

- ✓ 4 tablespoons cream cheese, reduced-fat but not fat free

- ✓ 4 tablespoons shredded parmesan cheese

- ✓ 1 (14-ounce) can preservative-free artichoke hearts OR 6- 8 artichoke hearts from a jar, drained and chopped

- ✓ 1 cup chopped grape or cherry tomatoes

- ✓ salt and pepper to taste

Instructions

- ✓ Place spinach, chicken broth, and chicken breasts in 4-quart slow cooker. Sprinkle with garlic, onion, and salt and pepper. Cover and cook on low for 6-8 hours, or on high from 4-6 hours.

- ✓ Just before serving, gently remove chicken breasts from the slow cooker and place on serving platters. Stir in cream cheese, parmesan cheese, and artichokes. Stir until creamy. Spoon sauce over chicken.

- ✓ Top with tomatoes. Sprinkle with extra parmesan cheese, if desired.

Snack:Paleo Friendly Meaty Veggie Roll Ups Smartpoints (Freestyle): 1

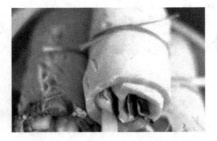

- ✓ Yields: 12 roll-ups

- ✓ Serving Size: 4-6 roll ups

- ✓ Calories: 71

- ✓ Total Fat: 2.0 g

- ✓ Saturated Fat: 0.6 g

- ✓ Trans Fat: 0 g

- ✓ Cholesterol: 29 mg

- ✓ Sodium: 27 mg

- ✓ Carbohydrates: 1.2 g

- ✓ Dietary Fiber: 0 g

- ✓ Sugars: 0.8 g

- ✓ Protein: 11.3g

✓ SmartPoints (Freestyle): 1

Ingredients

✓ 12 thick slices unprocessed deli meat, we recommend Boar's Head Brand

✓ 1 cup sliced vegetables

✓ 12 chives, optional

Instructions

✓ Place desired amount of vegetables on a piece of deli meat. Roll tightly, and if desired, use a chive to tie. Pack in a zip-top plastic bag or airtight container.

✓ Favorite Flavor Combinations:

✓ Roast beef with red bell pepper strips, carrot sticks, and cucumber slices with mustard for dipping.

✓ Chicken with apple slices, red cabbage, and pickle strips with Dijon mustard for dipping.

✓ Turkey with crumbled bacon and sliced avocado with salsa for dipping.

DAY 10 (24 SMARTPOINTS)

Breakfast: Overnight French Toast Casserole Smartpoints (Freestyle): 6

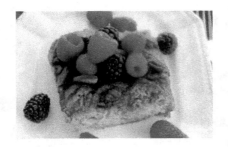

French toast is a rich, sweet breakfast treat. Our slow cooker twist is healthier and much easier to prepare than traditional French toast. Whether you are hosting several people at a brunch gathering or preparing a romantic breakfast in bed for two, this meal is sure to please.

✓ Yields: 10 Servings

✓ Serving: 2 Slices Bread

✓ Calories: 299

✓ Saturated Fat: 2 g

✓ Trans Fat: 0 g

✓ Cholesterol: 171 mg

✓ Sodium: 433 mg

✓ Total Carbohydrate: 38 g

✓ Dietary Fiber: 5 g

✓ Sugars: 14 g

✓ Protein: 15 g

✓ SmartPoints (Freestyle): 6

Ingredients

✓ 1 (13 ounce) loaf whole wheat French bread, sliced into 20 pieces

✓ 8 large eggs

✓ 2 cups low-fat milk, optional almond milk

✓ 1 teaspoon pure vanilla extract

✓ 1 teaspoon cinnamon

✓ 2 tablespoons coconut palm sugar or honey

✓ Topping

✓ 1/4 cup sucanat, optional coconut palm sugar or honey

✓ 1/2 cup minced pecans

✓ 1 teaspoon cinnamon

Instructions

✓ Lightly mist a 9" x 13" x 2" casserole dish with non-stick cooking spray. Arrange bread slices in two rows, slightly overlapping pieces. In a large mixing bowl, whisk together eggs, milk, vanilla, cinnamon and sucanat. Pour mixture over bread, making sure all bread is moist. Cover and refrigerate overnight.

✓ Preheat oven to 350 degrees. Combine topping ingredients, sprinkle evenly over the top of bread and bake 35 to 40 minutes, or until golden. Serve with fresh berries or a drizzle of pure maple syrup.

✓ NOTE: Whole Wheat French Bread can be purchased in the bakery section at most Walmart Super Centers, for about $1.00.

Lunch: Supermodel Superfood Salad Smartpoints (Freestyle): 6

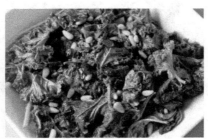

If it was possible for a vegetable to be sexy, then kale would be a supermodel. It is the "hottest" vegetable in town for a good reason. According to Web MD, one cup of kale provides 5 grams of fiber, 15% of calcium and B6, 40% magnesium, 180% vitamin A, 200% vitamin C and 1,020 % vitamin K. Those are impressive numbers toward the daily 100% of each needed, and all in 36 little calories per serving. It is also a good source of antioxidants like beta-carotene and folic acid. Move over spinach, no wonder kale is known as a "super food" and this supermodel superfood salad places it in the star position.

New salad recipes are always exciting. A fresh, new salad means exciting lunch for the next few days and a new party dish in your repertoire. Healthy salads are an even better find because you can eat them guilt-free and really feel as if you are filling up mid-day. The other great thing about superfood salads is sharing new, healthy foods with friends and family. When you bring this salad to your next get together, everyone will rave.

- ✓ Yields: 6 servings

- ✓ Calories: 162

- ✓ Total Fat: 13

- ✓ Saturated Fat: 2 g

- ✓ Trans Fat: 0 g

- ✓ Cholesterol: 35 mg

- ✓ Sodium: 16 mg

- ✓ Carbohydrates: 12 g

- ✓ Dietary Fiber: 2 g

- ✓ Sugars: 8 g

- ✓ Protein: 2 g

- ✓ SmartPoints (Freestyle): 6

Ingredients

- ✓ One head of kale

- ✓ 1/4 cup pine nuts

- ✓ 1/2 cup dried cranberries or currants

- ✓ Juice of 1 lemon

- ✓ 1/4 cup extra-virgin olive oil

- ✓ Pinch of kosher or sea salt

Instructions

- ✓ Remove and discard large stems of kale leaves. Coarsely chop kale leaves and add to a large serving bowl. Add pine nuts, dried cranberries or currants.

- ✓ Squeeze the juice of one lemon, drizzle with olive oil, and sprinkle salt, toss to combine.

- ✓ If desired, garnish with 1/4 cup freshly grated parmesan cheese.

Dinner: Asian Mango Chicken Stir-Fry Smartpoints (Freestyle): 8

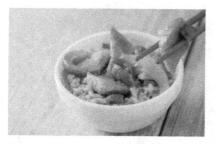

You will love how *q*uick and easy this Asian Mango Chicken Stir-Fry is. In less than 30 minutes, this recipe makes a delicious stir-fry dinner that your whole family will love. As usual, the SkinnyMs. team filled it with simple, whole ingredients. First, lean chicken breast, fresh peppers, onions, ginger, and mango make this dish fresh and filling. Finally, a tangy, sweet sauce made from orange juice and Asian seasonings makes this stir-fry oh so yummy. Skipping the takeout menu has never been so easy.

Our mango chicken stir-fry is light in calories, high in protein, while packing in delicious flavor. And because it's such a healthy version of a classic Asian dish, we're sure you'll want it on your menu rotation. To keep it even lighter, serve it over brown rice!

✓ Yields: 5 servings

✓ Serving Size: 1 cup

✓ Calories: 225

✓ Total Fat: 6g

- ✓ Saturated Fat: 1g

- ✓ Trans Fat: 0g

- ✓ Cholesterol: 48mg

- ✓ Sodium: 601mg

- ✓ Carbohydrates: 28g

- ✓ Fiber: 4g

- ✓ Sugar: 21g

- ✓ Protein: 17g

- ✓ SmartPoints (Freestyle): 8

Ingredients

- ✓ 1 tablespoon olive oil

- ✓ 4 boneless, skinless chicken breasts, sliced

- ✓ 1 small onion, sliced

- ✓ 1 red pepper, sliced

- ✓ 1 green pepper, sliced

- ✓ 2 mangos, peeled and sliced

- ✓ 1 teaspoon ground ginger

- ✓ 2 tablespoons low sodium chicken stock

- ✓ 2 tablespoons soy sauce

- ✓ 2 tablespoons rice vinegar

- ✓ 1 tablespoon pulp-free orange juice

- ✓ 2 tablespoons cornstarch

- ✓ 1 teaspoon black pepper

- ✓ 1/2 teaspoon kosher salt

Instructions

- ✓ Heat the oil over medium heat in a pan. Add the chicken and saute for 4 minutes. Remove chicken from the pan and add the onion. Cook until translucent, then add peppers. Cook 3 minutes then return the chicken. In a small bowl, whisk together the remaining ingredients and pour over the stir fry.

- ✓ Cook for 8 minutes, then serve over rice.

Snack: Skinny Bell Pepper Nacho Boats Smartpoints (Freestyle): 4

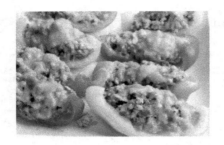

Sure- nachos taste delicious, but they probably don't rank high on the list of nutritious, wholesome recipes, especially when you're trying to eat healthy! However, you can satisfy your cravings for this classic Tex-Mex snack without worrying about your waistline by subbing in bell peppers for ordinary tortilla chips. This recipe for Bell Pepper Nacho Boats calls for delicious ingredients, like lean ground meat, savory spices, juicy salsa, and melted cheddar cheese.

✓ Yields: 18 boats

✓ Serving: 2 boats

✓ Calories: 145

✓ Total Fat: 9g

✓ Saturated Fat: 4g

✓ Trans Fat: 0g

✓ Cholesterol: 50mg

✓ Sodium: 293mg

✓ Carbohydrates: 4g

✓ Fiber: 1g

✓ Sugars: 2g

✓ Protein: 13g

✓ SmartPoints (Freestyle): 4

Ingredients

✓ 1 pound lean ground turkey

✓ 1 teaspoons chili powder

✓ 1 teaspoon cumin

✓ 1/2 teaspoon black pepper

✓ 1/4 teaspoon kosher or sea salt

✓ 3/4 cup salsa, no sugar added

✓ 1 cup grated cheddar cheese, reduced-fat

✓ 3 bell peppers

Instructions

✓ Remove seeds, core, and membrane from bell peppers then slice each one into 6 verticle pieces where they dip down. Set sliced bell peppers aside.

✓ Cook ground turkey over medium-high heat, breaking up as it cooks. Cook until the turkey loses it's pink color and is cooked through. Drain off any fat.

✓ Preheat oven to 375 degrees.

✓ Combine cooked turkey with spices and salsa. Evenly distribute mixture into the bell pepper boats, top with cheese.

✓ Bake on a parchment lined baking sheet for 10 minutes or until cheese is melted and peppers are hot. Optional ingredients: sliced Jalepeno peppers, diced avocado, fat-free Greek yogurt or sour cream, or sliced green onions.

✓ NOTE: If you prefer much softer bell peppers, add a few tablespoons water to the bottom of a large casserole dish, add filled nachos, cover tightly with foil and bake 15 minutes.

DAY 11 (20 SMARTPOINTS)

Breakfast: Flour-less Blueberry Oatmeal Muffins   Smart-Points (Freestyle): 5

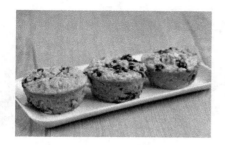

When I was growing up, my aunt had a gluten intolerance (before it was trendy.) At that time, producing *q*uality baked goods without flour was nearly impossible.

As a result, I saw years of brave gluten-free cakes, muffins, pie crusts, and quick breads meet their crumbly demise. One year, my aunt's attempt at a gluten-free carrot cake caved in on itself so badly it resembled a top hat. The top layer rising out of the deflated "brim" the bottom had crumbled into, we nicknamed it "the hat cake."

Much to my aunt's chagrin, that name lives on to this day.

✓ Yields: 1 dozen muffins

✓ Serving Size: 1 muffin

✓ Calories: 122

✓ Total Fat: 4g

✓ Saturated Fat: 2g

✓ Trans Fat: 0g

✓ Cholesterol: 16mg

✓ Sodium: 108mg

✓ Carbohydrates: 19g

✓ Fiber: 2g

✓ Sugar: 7g Protein: 3g

✓ SmartPoints (Freestyle): 5

Ingredients

✓ 2 1/2 cups old-fashioned rolled oats

✓ 1 1/2 cups almond milk

✓ 1 large egg, lightly beaten

✓ 1/3 cup pure maple syrup

✓ 2 tablespoons melted coconut oil

✓ 1 teaspoon vanilla extract

✓ 1 teaspoon ground cinnamon

✓ 1 teaspoon baking powder

✓ 1/4 teaspoon salt

✓ 1 teaspoon grated lemon zest

✓ 1 cup fresh blueberries

Instructions

✓ Combine the oats and almond milk in a large mixing bowl. Cover and refrigerate overnight.

✓ Preheat oven to 375 degrees. Spray a muffin tin with non-stick spray or line with muffin pan liners.

✓ Gently stir all ingredients into the soaked oats mixture. Spoon into the prepared muffin pan, filling about 3/4 full.

✓ Bake for about 20 minutes or until tops are golden. Serve warm.

Lunch: Chicken and Crisp Veggie Sandwich SmartPoints (Freestyle): 8

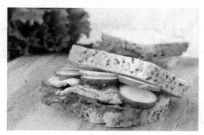

Chicken and Crisp Veggie SandwichSandwiches are a popular lunchtime staple around the world, and for good reason. In just one easy handful, you've combined complex carbohydrates with protein and veggies, with room for spreads and additional flavors that make your meal a joy to eat. And these days, sandwiches have gone upscale, with unique ingredient combinations and fun spreads. Everyone loves a good sandwich, and likely has a favorite or two at their go-to sandwich shop, but you can make a inventive, gourmet sandwich at home, saving yourself money, and scaling up your nutrition and healthy ingredients while scaling back the fat and calories in between some chain restaurant slices of bread.

Our Chicken and Crisp Veggie Sandwich is a healthy sandwich recipe with a complete balance of nutrition that will keep you fueled until dinnertime! We start with whole grain bread. Look for bread that contains whole grain as the first ingredient, or is labeled "7-grain" or "9-grain". These breads are full of whole, unprocessed grains that retain their dietary fiber content and nutritional value.

Then, add your chicken! Boneless, skinless chicken breasts are a healthy source of lean protein, and are easy on your wallet as well! Plus, radishes and cucumber provide antioxidants and a whole lot of crunch. And your spread can make or break this sandwich. Pour on the mayo, and you've got an uninspired and fatty sandwich. But get creative with healthier options like hummus and guacamole, and your tastebuds and waistline will thank you!

✓ *calculated with 1 tablespoon guacamole Yields: 1 sandwich/2 servings

✓ Serving Size: 1/2 sandwich

✓ Calories: 264

✓ Total Fat: 4 g

- ✓ Saturated Fat: 1 g

- ✓ Trans Fat: 0 g

- ✓ Cholesterol: 27 mg

- ✓ Sodium: 155 mg

- ✓ Carbohydrates: 41 g

- ✓ Dietary Fiber: 9 g

- ✓ Sugars: 13 g

- ✓ Protein: 21 g

- ✓ SmartPoints (Freestyle): 8

Ingredients

- ✓ 2 slices whole wheat or whole grain bread, toasted if desired

- ✓ 1 cooked (3 oz) boneless, skinless chicken breast

- ✓ 1 radish, thinly sliced

- ✓ 4- 5 slices cucumber

- ✓ 2 thin slices red onion (optional)

- ✓ 1 lettuce leaf, cut in half

✓ 1 tablespoon guacamole, hummus, or spread of choice

Instructions

✓ Assemble each sandwich by adding 1 tablespoon spread to each slice of bread, then topping with radish, cucumber, romaine lettuce and chicken breasts. Top with additional slice bread, flip over, cut in half, and serve.

Dinner: Baked Lemon Salmon And Asparagus Foil Pack Smartpoints (Freestyle): 2

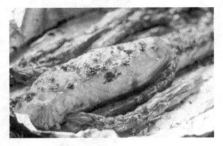

I've gushed about the wonders of salmon foil packs before, and I'll gush about them again. Salmon foil pack recipes make cooking, clean up, and portion control a cinch. Meanwhile, it's also a super versatile way of cooking. Oven or grill, a foil pack is an easy and delicious way to cook perfect, flavorful salmon. This baked lemon salmon and asparagus foil pack recipe makes a tasty and easy salmon dinner.

✓ Yields: 4 servings

✓ Calories: 386

✓ Total Fat: 26g

✓ Saturated Fat: 5g

✓ Trans Fat: 0g

✓ Cholesterol: 78mg

✓ Sodium: 558mg

✓ Carbohydrates: 7g

✓ Fiber: 3g

✓ Sugar: 3g

✓ Protein: 32g

✓ SmartPoints (Freestyle): 2

Ingredients

✓ 4 (4 to 6 ounce) filets salmon

✓ 1 pound fresh asparagus, about 1 inch of bottom ends trimmed off

✓ 1 teaspoon Kosher salt

✓ 1/2 teaspoon ground black pepper

✓ 2 tablespoons olive oil

- ✓ 1/4 cup fresh lemon juice

- ✓ 1 tablespoon fresh thyme, chopped

- ✓ 2 tablespoons fresh parsley, chopped

- ✓ 2 tablespoons lemon zest

Instructions

- ✓ Preheat the oven to 400 degrees.

- ✓ Lay 4 large sheets of foil on a flat surface and spray with nonstick spray. Divide the asparagus between each of the packets and lay in a single layer side by side. Season with half the salt and pepper.

- ✓ Place a salmon filet on top of each bed of asparagus. Drizzle with olive oil, lemon juice, thyme, and the remaining salt and pepper. Carefully fold up each side of the foil sheets to create a packet around the salmon and place in a single layer on a baking sheet. Bake for 15 minutes.

- ✓ Remove from the oven and carefully open each packet, be cautious of the steam released once opened! Sprinkle lemon zest and parsley on top. Serve and enjoy!

- ✓ Option: Try this recipe on the grill instead of in the oven for extra flavor!

Snack: Almond Butter And Banana Sandwiches Smartpoints (Freestyle): 5

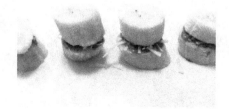

Who doesn't love a yummy snack?... Well if you're a snack lover like me, I've got the perfect snack for you!

These delicious and healthy little treats make for a great snack, dessert or part of any meal, and the best part? Almond Butter and Banana Sandwiches are super easy to make.

Bananas are a good source of potassium, an electrolyte that's key for proper muscle function and relaxation, and is also important for promoting balanced blood pressure. Potassium is also a key nutrient for hydration and fluid balance too.

Although bananas often get a bad wrap because they're higher in sugar than some other fruits, they do contain key nutrients like potassium, and they also contain prebiotics. Prebiotics are key nutrients because they act as food for healthy gut bacteria called probiotics (other sources of prebiotics include asparagus, garlic, onions, cabbage, beans, and bran). Healthy gut bacteria is key for weight management, insulin regulation and more.

✓ Yields: 2 servings

✓ Calories: 114

✓ Total Fat: 6g

✓ Saturated Fat: 1g

✓ Trans Fat: 0g

✓ Cholesterol: 0mg

✓ Sodium: 2mg

✓ Carbohydrates: 16g

✓ Fiber: 3g | Sugars: 8g

✓ Protein: 2g

✓ SmartPoints (Freestyle): 5

Ingredients

✓ 1 banana, sliced

✓ 1 Tbsp natural almond butter (enough for a dab in each sandwich)

✓ 1 Tbsp coconut flakes, unsweetened and no sulfites

✓ 1 Tbsp cacao nibs, (optional)

✓ Dash of cinnamon, (optional)

✓ Add a dash of cinnamon to each bite before closing the sandwich with 1-2 granules himalayan sea salt to each (optional)

Instructions

✓ Peel and slice the banana. Add almond butter and coconut along with other ingredients on 4-5 of the 8-10 slices.

✓ Close the sandwiches, and place the sandwiches on a plate or cookie sheet and place into the freezer. Allow the sandwiches to set for 20-30 minutes (or more), then serve and enjoy!

DAY 12 (22 SMARTPOINTS)

Breakfast: Tomato, Ham, And Poached Egg English Muffin Smartpoints (Freestyle): 6

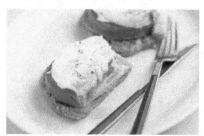

Every time we go out to breakfast, my boyfriend grapples with a deep, emotional decision: sweet or savory?

It's an age old breakfast dilemma. While this versatility in flavor palettes is part of what makes breakfast so amazing, it can also make for some serious decision-making struggles.

A committed sweet tooth, I can usually avoid this mental agony. Sure, an egg skillet or breakfast burrito may catch my eye. But ultimately, I always go straight for the sweet stuff—towers of pancakes, massive Belgian waffles, or stuffed French toast. As long as I can drench it in maple syrup, I'm there. Sure, there's plenty of variety out there when it comes to breakfast dishes. But am I really going to pass up the opportunity to start my day with a meal that is totally acceptable to top with whipped cream? Not a chance.

The only thing that's ever come between me and a giant plate of fluffy, sugary breakfast goodness? Eggs Benedict.

- ✓ Yields: 4 servings

- ✓ Calories: 209

- ✓ Total Fat: 11g

- ✓ Saturated Fat: 3g

- ✓ Trans Fat: 0g

- ✓ Cholesterol: 176mg

- ✓ Sodium: 503mg

- ✓ Carbohydrates: 16g

- ✓ Fiber: 3g

- ✓ Sugar: 4g

✓ Protein: 13g

✓ SmartPoints (Freestyle): 6

Ingredients

✓ 3 teaspoons olive oil

✓ 1 tomato, cut into 4 thick circle slices

✓ 4 slices low-sodium ham

✓ 2 whole wheat English muffins, cut in half

✓ 4 eggs, poached

✓ 1/4 teaspoon coarse ground black pepper

Instructions

✓ Heat 2 teaspoons of the olive oil in a skillet on medium heat. Once hot add the tomatoes and the ham and cook until ham is golden brown on each side and tomatoes are slightly soft.

✓ Place the ham on the English muffin and top with a tomato. Place the poached egg on top. Drizzle with the remaining teaspoon of olive oil and sprinkle with the coarse ground black pepper. Enjoy!

Lunch: Clean Eating Nut Butter And Jam Sandwich Smartpoints (Freestyle): 6

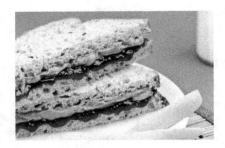

Just thinking about the peanut butter and jelly sandwiches your parents used to make for you as a child probably has you hankering for a bite of crunchy nut butter sweetened with ooey gooey fruit jam. Putting these two ingredients together inside a sandwich is the definition of comfort food. But traditionally, the peanut butter and jelly sandwiches of our youth were likely loaded with peanut butter packed with preservatives and jelly made with added refined sugar. Make a clean eating PB&J with our Clean Eating Nut Butter and Jam Sandwich.

The key to making a clean eating sandwich with nut butter and jam is to choose your ingredients wisely. Look for a peanut butter, almond butter, or hazelnut butter made with all natural ingredients, free of added sugars and preservatives. When choosing a jam, look for an organic label with no added sugar. So many jellies and jams are packed with added sweeteners, but we like a fruit jam that derives its sweetness from the fruit itself. And choose a whole grain bread. The first ingredient in your loaf should be whole grains, and if you see ingredients such as oats, flax, barley, hemp seeds, and dates, then you know you've got a healthy slice of bread. Whole grain bread is full of fiber and nutrients, and is a complex carbohydrate that's 100% guilt-free.

- ✓ Yield: 1 sandwich, 2 servings

- ✓ Serving Size: 1/2 sandwich

- ✓ Calories: 187

- ✓ Total Fat: 9 g

- ✓ Saturated Fat: 1 g

- ✓ Trans Fat: 0 g

- ✓ Cholesterol: 0 mg

- ✓ Sodium: 115 mg

- ✓ Carbohydrates: 22 g

- ✓ Dietary Fiber: 4 g

- ✓ Sugars: 6 g

- ✓ Protein: 8 g

- ✓ SmartPoints (Freestyle): 6

Ingredients
- ✓ 2 tablespoons of your favorite clean eating nut butter (store bought or homemade

- ✓ 1 tablespoon Polaner All Fruit Spread of choice or other fruit sweetened jam

- ✓ 2 slices whole wheat or whole grain sandwich bread

Instructions

- ✓ Spread the nut butter on one slice of bread. Spread the jam on the other slice of bread. Put both pieces together, slice in half, and enjoy!

Dinner: One Pot Turkey and Mediterranean Quinoa SmartPoints (Freestyle): 4

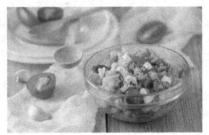

If you appreciate Mediterranean flavors, you'll love our One Pot Turkey Sausage and Mediterranean Quinoa. We've taken nitrate-free turkey sausage and combined it with quinoa, so it's a healthy, nutrient-rich meal. Tomatoes and spinach add tons of vitamins, while feta cheese adds a Mediterranean flair. And since it uses just one dish, you'll want to make it again and again.

It's also easy to customize. For a more decidedly Mediterranean flavor, you can use turkey Italian sausage instead, and add a sprinkling of herbs like oregano or basil. The choices are endless!

But whatever you do, don't skimp on the feta. That briny flavor really gives the dish a nice salty pop!

- ✓ Yields: 4 servings

- ✓ Servings Size: 1 cup

- ✓ Calories: 117

- ✓ Total Fat: 8g

- ✓ Saturated Fat: 3g

- ✓ Trans Fat: 0g

- ✓ Cholesterol: 17mg

- ✓ Sodium: 455mg

- ✓ Carbohydrates: 8g

- ✓ Fiber: 3g

- ✓ Sugar: 4g

- ✓ Protein: 5g

- ✓ SmartPoints (Freestyle): 4

Ingredients
- ✓ 1 tablespoon extra virgin olive oil

- ✓ 2 cups nitrate free turkey rope sausage, cut into 1 inch chunks

- ✓ 2 clove garlic, minced

- ✓ 1 small yellow onion, cut into strips

- ✓ 1 cup low sodium chicken broth

- ✓ 1 (14 ounce) can diced tomatoes

- ✓ 1/2 teaspoon Kosher salt

- ✓ 1 1/2 cups *q*uinoa, rinsed in cool water

- ✓ 2 cups spinach, chopped

- ✓ 1/2 cup low fat feta cheese, crumbled

Instructions

- ✓ In large skillet, heat oil on medium heat. Once hot, add turkey sausage, garlic, and onion. Cook until onion begins to soften. Stir in broth, tomatoes, salt, and *q*uinoa. Bring to a boil and reduce to a simmer and add spinach. Continue to simmer, stirring occasionally to prevent *q*uinoa from sticking, until broth is absorbed. Spoon into serving bowls and sprinkle with feta. Enjoy!

Snack: Cranberry Pumpkin Seed Granola Smartpoints (Freestyle): 6

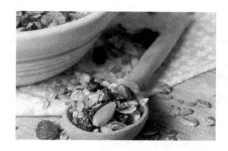

We love granola for breakfast. It is delicious when paired with Greek yogurt, served with almond milk and fresh fruit, or even just enjoyed plain! Making homemade Cranberry Granola may sound a little intimidating, but it truly is *q*uite easy. With just a little stirring and baking time, you can save quite a bit of money by not buying granola at the store.

The combinations for granola recipes are endless, but we really enjoy Cranberry Pumpkin Seed Granola in colder months. The color of the green pumpkin seeds and red cranberries truly get us in a festive mood!

✓ Yields: 16-18 servings

✓ Serving Size: 1/2 cup

✓ Calories: 189

✓ Total Fat: 9.8 g

✓ Saturated Fat: 1.4 g

✓ Trans Fat: 0 g

- ✓ Cholesterol: 0 mg

- ✓ Sodium: 5 mg

- ✓ Carbohydrates: 20.8 g

- ✓ Dietary Fiber: 4.0 g

- ✓ Sugars: 8.2 g

- ✓ Protein: 5.4 g

- ✓ SmartPoints (Freestyle): 6

Ingredients

- ✓ 4 cups rolled oats

- ✓ 1 cup raw pumpkin seeds

- ✓ ½ cup flax seed

- ✓ ¼ cup sesame seeds

- ✓ 3 teaspoons cinnamon

- ✓ 1/3 cup honey

- ✓ 1/4 cup pure maple syrup

- ✓ 1/4 cup sunflower oil

- ✓ 1 tsp vanilla

✓ 1 cup dried cranberries, (optional dried cherries, apricots or raisins)

Instructions

✓ Preheat oven to 250 degrees Fahrenheit and prepare 2 baking sheets with parchment paper.

✓ In a large bowl, gently mix the oats, pumpkin seeds, flax, sesame and cinnamon. To this mixture add the honey, syrup, oil, and vanilla and stir until well-combined.

✓ Spread the mixture on the baking sheets and cook for 60 -75 minutes. To achieve and even color on the granola while baking, stir every 15 minutes.

✓ Remove granola and allow to cool before adding the dried cranberries. Store in an air-tight container.

DAY 13 (26 SMARTPOINTS)

Breakfast: Slow Cooker Sweet Potato Oatmeal Smartpoints (Freestyle): 6

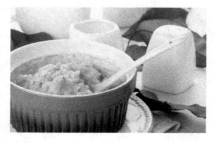

Looking for a prefect pre-workout meal that provides tons of lasting energy? Look no further! Sweet Potato Oatmeal is comprised of complex carbs that provides lasting energy due to high fiber content, and tons of nutrients. Superfood sweet potato lends a sweet, earthy flavor to this easily prepared breakfast. Combine ingredients in your slow cooker and sit back while your delicious, energizing meal simmers away!

NOTE: The carbohydrates in this recipe are complex carbs that are stored and used as energy that lasts all day and are found primarily in the oats and sweet potato. Simple carbs cause an immediate spike in blood sugar and can be found in foods like pastries and candy.

✓ Servings: 6

✓ Serving Size: 1 cup

✓ Calories: 164

✓ Total Fat: 3 g

✓ Saturated Fats: 1 g

✓ Trans Fats: 0 g

✓ Cholesterol: 3 mg

✓ Sodium: 56 mg

✓ Carbohydrates: 45 g

- ✓ Dietary Fiber: 5 g

- ✓ Sugars: 14 g

- ✓ Protein: 8 g

- ✓ SmartPoints (Freestyle): 6

Ingredients

- ✓ 1 cup steel cut oats

- ✓ 2 cups low-fat milk

- ✓ 2 cups water

- ✓ 1 cup grated sweet potato, or 1/2 cup cooked and mashed sweet potato

- ✓ 2 tablespoons unrefined sweetener, more or less to taste, I used coconut palm sugar. Other options: sucanat, honey or 100% pure maple syrup

- ✓ Kosher or sea salt to taste

- ✓ 1/2 teaspoon cinnamon

- ✓ 1 teaspoon pumpkin pie spice

Instructions

✓ Combine all ingredients in the slow cooker, cover and cook on low 2 to 2 1/2 hours, or until desired consistency is reached. Recommend 4-5 *q*uart slow cooker.

✓ If desired, add diced nuts and raisins.

STOVE TOP METHOD: Add all ingredients to a medium saucepan, bring to a boil, reduce heat to a simmer and cook approximately 20 - 25 minutes, or until desired consistency has been reached.

Lunch: Chickpea And Tomato Salad Smartpoints (Freestyle): 5

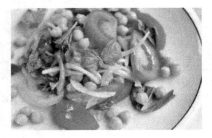

What exactly is a chickpea, anyway?

This thought usually crosses my mind at some point whenever I encounter chickpeas. So before we dive into this Simple Chickpea Salad recipe, I thought it might help to get some background. When you think about it, chickpeas are a pretty unique food, as far as canned goods go. Not a vegetable, not a grain, and certainly neither chick nor pea, it can be hard to define what exactly a chickpea is.

Now, please don't read my confusion as criticism. I absolutely love chickpeas, in all their forms. Give them to me in a salad, mashed into hummus, or ground into falafel. I show up for chickpeas all day long. They've got a one of a kind texture and a subtle earthy flavor that makes them a versatile complement to all kinds of meals and snacks.

That said, my love for chickpeas alone has never really satisfied my curiosity about what exactly they are. If anything, it's only discouraged me from finding out. I usually just figure I like them enough that it doesn't really matter what they are.

Today, for your benefit and my own, I have done some laborious Googling to finally shed light on this mystery. (Drumroll please...)

Turns out, chickpeas are a legume. If that information isn't helpful, some other notable legumes include:

✓ Beans

✓ Lentils

✓ Soybeans

✓ Peas (So I guess the "pea" part of chickpea isn't totally misleading after all.)

Peanuts ("Did you know that peanuts aren't nuts?" is always a quality fun fact to have up your sleeve.)

- ✓ Yields: 6 servings

- ✓ Serving Size: 1/2 cup

- ✓ Calories: 144

- ✓ Total Fat: 4g

- ✓ Saturated Fat: 0g

- ✓ Trans Fat: 0g

- ✓ Cholesterol: 0mg

- ✓ Sodium: 330mg

- ✓ Carbohydrates: 22g

- ✓ Fiber: 6g

- ✓ Sugar: 7g

- ✓ Protein: 6g

- ✓ SmartPoints (Freestyle): 1

Ingredients
- ✓ 1 (14 ounce) can chickpeas drained and rinced

- ✓ 1/4 cup basil leaves, roughly chopped

- ✓ 1 tablespoon olive oil

✓ 1 small yellow onion, sliced thin

✓ 6 large tomatoes, sliced into 1/2 inch thick wedges

✓ 1/2 teaspoon Kosher salt

✓ 1 tablespoon dark balsamic vinegar

Instructions

✓ In a large bowl, combine all ingredients and toss well ensuring all ingredients are coating in the oil and vinegar. Let rest, covered, in the refrigerator for 20 minutes. Toss before serving and enjoy!

Dinner: Easy Chicken Bruschetta Casserole Smartpoints (Freestyle): 8

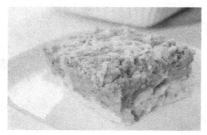

You know what I love about bruschetta? You get a little bit of everything. The experience starts with a crunchy piece of bread, but then it blooms into something special once you bite into those saucy tomatoes and fresh herbs. You get a burst of sweet flavor and a punch of savoriness. It's a perfect one-bite, but it's not really a dish appropriate for dinner. So we made a dinner version: this healthy chicken bruschetta casserole. There's a lot to celebrate with this one-pan dish. Lean chicken breast filets provide a ton of protein while also being super easy to cook. The chicken is seasoned with garlic, black pepper, and oregano – the same flavors on my favorite appetizer! And then there's the topping. Oh, that delicious breadcrumb topping.

You might think that breadcrumbs are breadcrumbs – but I'd have to disagree. When we combine them with chicken broth and diced tomatoes, the dry crumbs become hydrated and the whole thing transforms into a savory topping. Once they bake up over the seasoned chicken, you end up with an upside-down piece of bruschetta. Perfect!

- ✓ Yields: 6 cups

- ✓ Serving Size: 1 cup

- ✓ Calories: 463

- ✓ Total Fat: 18g

- ✓ Saturated Fat: 6g

- ✓ Trans Fat: 0g

- ✓ Cholesterol: 88mg

- ✓ Sodium: 967mg

- ✓ Carbohydrates: 38g

✓ Fiber: 4g

✓ Sugar: 5g

✓ Protein: 36g

✓ SmartPoints (Freestyle): 8

Ingredients

✓ 2 1/2 cups herb seasoned bread crumbs (we used Pepperidge Farm's Herb Seasoned stuffing mix)

✓ 1/2 cup fat-free chicken broth (optional water)

✓ 1 (15-ounce) can petit diced tomatoes

✓ 1.5 pounds chicken breast filets, cut into small bite size pieces

✓ 1/2 teaspoon garlic powder

✓ 1/2 teaspoon black pepper

✓ 1/2 teaspoon salt

✓ 1 1/2 teaspoons dried oregano

✓ 1 cup part-skim mozzarella

Instructions

✓ Preheat oven to 400 degrees.

✓ In a mixing bowl combine bread crumbs, chicken broth, and diced tomatoes with liquid, set aside.

✓ In a 9 x 13-inch casserole pan add chicken pieces, garlic powder, pepper, salt, oregano, and 3/4 cup cheese, toss to combine.

✓ Add bread crumb mixture and spread evenly over chicken. Sprinkle with the remaining cheese.

✓ Bake for 35 minutes, or until chicken is done.

Snack: Chocolate Peanut Butter Protein Smoothie Smartpoints (Freestyle): 7

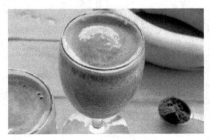

The combination of chocolate and peanut butter makes a smoothie even the youngest member of the family will devour. Cocoa powder and peanut butter are crowd-pleasers, while banana and Greek yogurt add potassium and protein to this sweet, satisfying, and nutritious smoothie.

✓ *calculated with natural peanut butter and coconut palm sugar Yields: 3 servings

- ✓ Serving Size: 1 cup

- ✓ Calories: 214

- ✓ Total Fat: 11 g

- ✓ Saturated Fat: 0 g

- ✓ Trans Fat: 0 g

- ✓ Cholesterol: 5

- ✓ Carbohydrates: 22 g

- ✓ Sodium: 57 mg

- ✓ Dietary Fiber: 4 g

- ✓ Sugars: 10 g

- ✓ Protein: 10 g

- ✓ SmartPoints (Freestyle): 7

Ingredients

- ✓ 2 tablespoons cocoa powder

- ✓ 3 tablespoons natural peanut butter (optional, organic Powdered Peanut Butter which is much lower in fat & calories than regular peanut butter.)

- ✓ 1 cup low-fat milk, (optional, almond or soy milk)

- ✓ 1 frozen banana, pre-sliced

- ✓ 1/2 cup plain Greek yogurt, fat-free

- ✓ 2 tablespoons coconut palm sugar, honey is optional

- ✓ 1/2 teaspoon pure vanilla extract

- ✓ ice as needed

Instructions

- ✓ Combine all ingredients in a blender and blend until smooth. Add ice according to desired thickness.

CONCLUSION

Weight Watchers research has come up with overwhelmingly favorable findings about the reasonable laws of the company, and the fresh program is even more in line with what nutritionists are recommending.

Other studies have discovered that members of Weight Watchers also tend to reduce their likelihood of heart disease and blood pressure, as it has also been shown to do exercise and weight loss in particular.

So while it may be surprising that Weight Watchers doesn't consider how much weight members want to spend on the scheme, it's actually a pretty good thing, scientifically.

Do Not Go Yet; One Last Thing To Do

If you enjoyed this book or found it useful I'd be very grateful if you'd post a short review on Amazon. Your support really does make a difference and I read all the reviews personally so I can get your feedback and make this book even better.

Thanks again for your support!